Dying

Without

Crying

J.I. Willett

"In simple words, the author opens a vista of complex human emotions. We are brought to the edge of life while enveloped in a look back moment that attempts to provide meaning to our overall existence.

The reader is overwhelmed by the descriptive examples of human interaction that are used to exemplify the many views and fears we each confront when facing the great mystery of death. The book contains many instructive tools, created through meaningful vignettes to help us handle and make sense of the death of loved ones as well help us face our own mortality. Moreover, the book provides a spiritual reassurance that death is not the end. Regardless of our own religious beliefs and without imposing the author's views upon the reader, Ms. Willett provides us with a certain comfort about the spiritual life after death that many religions fail to fully explore. "

~ ROBERT DENNIS

M.D., F.A.A.O.S., C.I.M.E.; And author, Informed Health Plan Act of 2017

"*Perhaps because I have been a caregiver profession-ally for over 30 years, and also for family members, I really like this book. The author clearly has experience in the field from the details given. There is an overriding sense of reality in the work - that is 'no one gets out of this world alive' -without being depressing or unrealis-tically spiritual. Impending death hurts but does NOT have to be a battle lost, neither is it a picnic in the park for all concerned.*

The book provides useful, actionable tips for those with little experience in this realm of life. Dignity, the right to make decisions, the right to be treated as a living per-son by all, medical professionals, family, friends and others, is key to this challenging time. This work is a roadmap to help the reader accomplish that."

~ DENNIS McGEEHAN

Professional Healthcare Provider

"In her book, "Dying without Crying," J.I. Willett has truly captured the struggles and triumphs of those dealing with terminal illness. Her book is a beautiful, concise guide for both those who are terminally ill and those caring for them. It reiterates the need for all of us to remember to love and respect each other, and live each day to its fullest! "

~ CAROL A. JOHNSON

LCSW, Geriatric Care Manager

"I was truly moved by this book! From the first sentence to the last poem, "Dying Without Crying" will take you on a journey not just through the author's experiences but the common experience of facing death with dignity and the sometimes difficult emotions and circumstances that accompany it. Just like the Resurrection of Jesus, Janice's experiences will bring you hope that even in death there can be room for new life; and that the end-of-life journey is really just preparation for the glorious new adventure that waits for us beyond the veil. This book will help you to "pack your bags" or help another do the same; and leave this life surrounded by

love, set free from regret, and ready to enter the waiting arms of a compassionate Father".

~ REV. BRUCE J. WOOD

Lead Pastor First Baptist Church, Hightstown, NJ

"I loved your book. You courageously approached a difficult subject matter, and have slammed the ball out of the park! You have created a practical, yet compassionate, source of comfort to those in need. God bless you for perpetuating one's dignity in their transition, while lessening the heartbreak of their loved ones. No one gives us a book on how to live when we come into this world, but you have surely given us a book on how to move on to the next world."

~ JOHN J. GRANDE

CFP, Board member -Tissue Banks International

"The work is "book-ended" by two magnificent poems that convey the author's essential message very well. Both are very simple poems that indicate that death need not be viewed as a total end. When I read the title, I assumed the "without crying" referred to the person facing a near-term death; but it quickly became obvious that it also referred to the loved ones on the journey with them. The writing is very clear, as is the message. After reading the Table of Contents, I was very much interested in reading the whole book"

~ THOMAS E. PORTER

Author, Is a Catholic A Christian?

In loving memory of family and friends

who have travelled down the road before me.

My thanks to all those involved

during the writing of this book;

especially my forever friend, Pamela H. Zuczek,

for being my sounding board and best critic.

I acknowledge with love and appreciation Lona Mae Fowler, who encouraged me to write this book. I met Lona approximately 30 years before her passing from breast cancer in August of 2009.

When Lona was diagnosed with breast cancer, modern medicine intervened with the list of what-to-do. Although Lona's preference was to just 'be', she followed the medical dictates, despite failing to improve during these procedures and processes. For some, the medical agenda is a miracle and for others life becomes more painful and complicated.

Throughout the years, Lona taught me that friendships are like gardens and friends the gardeners. We need to water and nurture friendships with respect and love in order for them to come into full bloom.

Good friends are our cheerleaders, listeners, lifesavers, shoulders to lean on, jokesters and singers of songs. They laugh together, cry together, shout and rejoice together. Through faith they grow the ability to share God's blessings and wisdom. I have learned that friends can become "family," and family can become friends.

Contents

Dying Without Crying is an informative, easy, quick read containing core information for caregivers and care receivers on setting boundaries and having a voice during the final journey in this life.

Although there are many "how-to" books that offer methodical approaches and are timely to read, this compact book offers a big message with complete simplicity.

The information contained herein is based on personal experiences during the last phases of life with my grandmother, parents, an uncle and aunt, and several friends - many of whom I had the privilege to be with during their passing.

Through this book I hope to help you find encouragement to be strong, to find and use your voice and intuition, to hold your head high, stay firm in your convictions and know there is not an end - it is another beginning.

My goal is to help others communicate effectively and peacefully during difficult situations; to maintain grace and dignity so in the end, rather

than grieve, we can celebrate our everlasting con-
nections.

Remember, we are all travelling down the same
road; we just arrive at different times.

What Is Dying?

I am standing on the sea shore.

A ship at my side spreads her

white sails in the morning breeze

and starts for the blue ocean.

She is an object of beauty and I

stand and watch her until at last

she fades on the horizon.

Then someone at my side says

There, she has gone -

Gone where?

Gone from my sight - that is all

She is just as large in the mast,

hull and spars as she was

when she left my side....

The diminished size

and total loss of sight

is in me and not in her,

and just at the moment when

someone by my side says

"She is gone"

others take up the glad shout

"Here she comes!"

And that is dying.

~ Bishop Charles Henry Brent (1862-1929)

Know Thyself

Knowing one is going to die is not for the weak-hearted, it becomes an act of courage. Despite our fears, we must begin to search within ourselves to locate the depths of our inner voice, our soul, our Godliness.

We have within ourselves the ability to move beyond our fears, whether we accept any medical procedures or contradict them as being unsuitable for ourselves. We need to assess if the disease is terminal and if medical procedures may only pro-long time but not provide for a quality of time ... if the choice is worth the suffering or pain.

I am the captain

of my ship.

I am the captain of my ship. No one else knows how to adjust my sails but me.

Only I know when the stormy weather
is approaching, or the swells calm down.
Only I know how much water I can hold
before I start bailing out. Only I can see
the red in the sky from the setting sun or
the rain filled clouds of morning. I have
to say to myself take heed, take control,
for this is MY journey, no one else's. I
must make it my business to be in charge
and control of MY destiny.

Doctors are human, just like you and me. They do their best with their medical knowledge and training. It's okay to speak of our needs and desires, our decisions of tests, medicines and care. It really is okay. It is important to express your feelings, even if they are contrary to recommendations. The physicians need to know how you feel. Remember ... you and your medical providers should be working in unison for an agreed upon anticipated outcome.

Too many times we forget to be proactive in allowing our bodies' natural self-healing mechanisms to engage. In addition to medicine, utilize the numerous books and videos readily available that focus on guided meditations, which can activate the deep healing powers only we can create within our bodies.

And … never underestimate the power of prayer! Prayer to assist you in making sound decisions, prayer for the medical personnel treating you, prayer for physical healing, and prayer for spiritual nourishment.

What Kind Of Soldier Do We Want To Be?

When we face the unexpected news of a terminal illness, we will experience many emotions ... each to a different degree. We may be angry. We may be sad. We may cry. We may bes scared. We may feel like breaking something and screaming. We may experience self-pity, regrets. Some of these we can change, and some we may not.

Dealing with so many emotions is a difficult process, and only we can tame them. Lona envisioned herself as a soldier, being in the forefront, setting an example for those she would be leaving behind. She knew her example would serve others for their transition to the afterlife. She wore her uniform of bravery and marched through her fears. Through this valiant march, she found her rhythm, which was ever changing ... daily, weekly, or at times moment by moment ... and continued her journey as bravely as possible.

Remember ... we all travel down the same road; we just arrive at different times. I feel peace knowing that Lona is leading the way. She, by example, showed me that there is nothing to fear when my time comes.

And know, please listen carefully ... KNOW that one of the most troublesome aspects of this journey may not be with you, it may be with someone else. It may be people that are not so strong. It may be people who are self-seeking and not in your presence for positive reasons. Don't allow them to weaken the good fight you've begun. Never feel guilty saying 'no' to visits and phone calls. As much as possible, surround yourself with people who support your choices.

This is your

journey.

This is your journey. You need to have your mantra, "I will do the best I can for as long as I can. I am the captain of my ship."

When my son was about five years old we were driving past our neighbor's house on a dark rainy Saturday morning. Her covered body was being placed in an ambulance and I began to cry. My son questioned what was happening and why I was crying. When I told him he replied, "But does SHE know she's dead?"

That's what it's all about. Life is continuous movement - movement from one plane to another - from one reality to another. Only our physical body ceases, not our soul, our essence, our being.

Let me ask you, how many people do we know that are alive, yet dead inside?

Stay In The Now

L earn to live in the present moment. The present is now, not five minutes ago, not in ten minutes, not last year or next month ... *now*.

We can control *now*. The past is behind us and the future is yet to come. If we worry about the past, we cannot be in the present. We have no control over the future, only the present.

> *By changing our attitudes, we change the present.*

By changing our attitudes, we change the present. It's who you are right now that matters! Go with it, be it, feel it, write about it, tell about it ... just be who you are right now! If you are angry, go with it. If you are happy, go with it. Whatever you are right now, go with it, accept it, be it and get through it.

As to whatever goes on in the rest of the world, we need to be kind and thoughtful. Do not get caught up in others' self-imposed importance. Now is our time. Not the time of the visitor who has come not to assist you, but to drain you. We can learn to say "now is not a good time for a visit." Why? Because we control "*now.*" We want our time with visitors and friends to be valuable. We want to enjoy our visits and enrich each other's lives with our stories, experiences, and thoughts.

We need to think about all the things we regret not having done and make a list. Consider how many, if not all, of the items you can do *now.* Skydive? Sail? Fish? A vacation? Visit a distant friend or relative? Write a book? See a Broadway show? The events can be endless. Now is the time. Every day becomes *now.* Some days we may feel more energetic than others; so we pick something on the list that can be fulfilled according to how we feel *now.*

We should not feel guilty about having fun, pleasure, or enjoyment ... we deserve it! Surely there will be the cynical 'friends' who will say we are just too ill or unrealistic; in other words, imposing their judgments in an effort for us to feel guilty for having fun while dying.

We shouldn't have to be afraid to live while we are dying. We should be afraid of dying while we should be living.

Patience, My Friend, Patience

There are two types of caregivers. The first type consists of individuals who provide home health care … such as family, friends and medically trained personnel. The second type is a medical institution or caregiving facility such as a hospital, assisted living facility or nursing home.

For home care we first create a plan that is viable for the patient and caregiver(s). Set up a meeting to create a business plan to outline the involved parties' needs and expectations. Discuss what needs are required on an hourly, daily or weekly basis. Tasks that are routine, such as the receiver needs cups, plates and silverware every morning, can be prepared each evening by the caregiver. These small gestures eliminate the need for the patient to begin to feel badly to ask for the same items every morning, and the caregiver thinking 'here we go again with another request'. Plan that every morning at 8 am (or the prior evening) to set out the cups, plates and silverware.

Review everything you can think the patient might need. Certainly items can be added or deleted time to time, but the more routines you create, the more you will reduce the level of frustration for both parties. Do we need to set out vitamins, pills, washcloths and toothbrushes? On what day do we need to plan to do a load of laundry? How does the patient like the laundry done? What will be needed on a regular basis from the grocery store? Banking? Paying bills? Discuss which days and times are best for doctor appointments.

Have a list and calendar available for all parties involved. By doing this, the care receiver doesn't feel that he or she is a burden by constantly asking for something … and the caretaker doesn't feel overwhelmed by continual requests.

Allot about 15 minutes in the morning and 15 minutes later in the day for various unexpected tasks that may need to be done. The care receiver can write on a pad the extra things he or she thought of rather than continuously asking the receiver to handle extra needs if they are not emergent. Now the caregiver isn't feeling that every time they sit down, their name is being called.

We seem to forget the simplicity because it gets lost in the complexities that we, ourselves, create.

We seem to forget the simplicity because it gets lost in the complexities that we, ourselves, create.

As for the patient being cared for in a medical or care facility, there are some different situations to be addressed ... and usually best done with the supervisors for each shift. Be sure to provide each shift with a clear outline of what items were discussed and how they were agreed upon to be handled.

I have seen situations when meals were never delivered to a patient's room and the patient was unable to communicate it. I've also seen food brought in and set on the rolling tray table left too far for the patient to reach ... the server just puts it on the table tray where ever it sits in the room. The food then remains untouched for lack of access by the patient, later to be removed by the collection attendant who clearly sees the meal was untouched and the patient was incapable of accessing it. Day in and day out, many patients are ignored. They lack personal care, daily sustenance of food and water, human touch and kindnesses.

Unfortunately, there are also medical caregivers that believe all patients should be in diapers whether or not they are incontinent, to avoid the need to assist them in the bathroom.

I recall the first day of my aunt's stay in a nursing facility. She indicated she needed the bathroom. When I asked the nearby nurse for assistance, she calmly replied, "Just tell her to go in her diaper". What? In her diaper? My

Aunt was in total control of her bathroom habits. She didn't need a diaper; she needed assistance! How demeaning and demoralizing. I soon learned when my aunt was admitted they immediately put a diaper on her! She didn't have one on upon admittance and no one consulted with my aunt. They just put it on for the convenience of the staff. Dignity, people, dignity! Please! Yes, there is a shortage of staff in some facilities, but that doesn't mean a level of kindness, caring, respect and dignity has to be ignored.

On the other hand, when my aunt was in an assisted living facility the residents were in clean, neat outfits every morning. No pajamas. Everyone was well groomed; the ladies with make-up and lipstick. There were no bathroom related odors, and the level of care was impressive.

It is paramount to do thorough research when selecting a care facility. Take a walk through the halls and privately ask residents what they think about their level of care. Ask to have a meal in the dining room during scheduled mealtime to evaluate the service, taste and quality of the food. Notice if there are odors in the rooms and halls. Are the bathrooms clean? How well is the facility staffed? Do the residents appear alert, well nourished and neatly appareled? Is the general atmosphere one of despair or happiness? Lastly ... is it a place in which you would want to stay?

After the decision is made for where the patient will reside, caregivers PLEASE provide the receiver with what he or she needs - not what you think they need or what you are in the mood to provide. Treat the patient with the same respect and dignity that you would hope to receive for yourself.

We do care if there are stains on our clothes and they are wrinkled. We do care if our hair is dirty and our nails unkempt. We do want to be bathed and have an acceptable level of appearance for visitors and ourselves. Remember, although our bodies may be dying, our dignity is very much alive.

Who Needs A Martyr?

The dictionary defines a martyr as a person who displays or exaggerates their discomfort or distress in order to obtain sympathy or admiration.

Let's think about that. We can probably recall at least a handful of folks we've witnessed in the past month that would fit that description.

Now there will be some patients that feel they are cheated if they are not given large doses of medications and tests. It becomes part of their arsenal to challenge the other patients; the game of "whatever you have, I have worse."

It's like the decorations servers wear at some of the fast food chains - all the buttons and little medals on their uniforms - a hundred badges for the martyr.

Don't get caught up in that trap; either as being the martyr or defending ourselves against one. No need to participate in medical treatment competitions because the more power we give our situation and dwell on it, the more magnified our illness can become. Theaters of the mind, theaters of the body; we are what we think and become what we focus on.

Bottom line: We don't need medals. We need family, good friends, companionship, an acceptable level of care, and the best quality of life we can attain at any given time.

It's What Comes Out
Of It That Matters

Years ago I read a story about a man who happened upon a Monarch moth's cocoon. When he noticed the moth was desperately trying to squeeze its' way through the pin-size hole, the man decided to assist the moth by making the hole a little wider. The moth emerged easily; however, its' wings didn't function. Puzzled, the man later learned that what he felt the moth needed caused the moth to lose it's ability to fly. Had the moth squeezed through the tiny hole as God intended, the pressure would have pushed the moth's blood into its' wings to take to the air.

I believe there is a relationship between the experience of the Monarch and our lives. There are times we are struggling in the midst of transition, and often that "squeeze" will help us find our inner strength to rise above the experience. Feeling the squeeze causes us to change, which is a continuous process throughout our life. It may also allow us to evaluate if we, in fact, are squeezing the life out of ourself and others with our attitudes ... or allowing others to squeeze the life out of us.

Self-reflection at these times is important. Now is the opportunity to take our pain and suffering and examine it. Unleash any vines and thorns grown out of past experiences that have been constricting our hearts. It's time to forgive our self and others of wrong doings. Ask for forgiveness as well as bestow forgiveness, even if the other person does not ask. Forgiveness is a powerful tool that heals hearts and frees souls. Forgiveness mends friendships and families. Forgiveness eases pain and suffering. Forgiveness brings us closer to peace and holiness.

In the alternative, be aware of the impact of denying someone forgiveness. Before my uncle died, he repeatedly asked my mother to forgive him for an act of malice; and my mother repeatedly insisted it never happened. It was very clear that my uncle felt he couldn't move to the light until he made good on earth and this conversation created emotional conflict for him.

If someone asks to be forgiven, even if you truly can't recall the incident, graciously respond, "yes, I forgive you". If someone is having a difficult time saying what it is that they would like to be forgiven for, we need to let them know that we don't need the details. We only need to know they care enough to regret ever hurting us and we can just say, "it's okay, I forgive you".

Saying "I forgive you" and "please forgive me" are powerful statements, especially when saying good-bye. Everyone needs to be forgiven in order to fly.

Forgiveness leads to healing of our hearts and souls. Through the process of forgiveness we release negativity and begin a purification process that frees us. We become more spirited, more prepared, willing and peaceful to continue our journey forward.

It seems that when a person is at death's door all sins want to be forgiven. When they are not, the one passing is left tormented and struggling due to lack of closure. It is very sad when a person makes an effort to redeem oneself with another before leaving this world, and the other person won't grant it.

---

*Although we
cannot change the
past we can make
peace with it.*

Although we cannot change the past we can make peace with it.

Often it takes the darkest moments in our lives to go through the process of refining and purifying our spirit and heart in order to improve our emotional and spiritual journey. It's not always the healing of the body, but the healing of hearts and souls.

Remember, it's what comes out of the experience that matters.

No One Should Die Alone

We are not alone when we enter this world, nor should we be when we leave it.

If the opportunity permits, chose in advance the people you would like to surround yourself with at the time of final transition ... people who are encouraging and make you feel loved and safe.

This is your pilgrimage. In the end, no matter how many are with us, we take the final step alone.

This would be a good time to honor those who have passed before us; for those are the relationships we draw upon to help us embrace both life and death. They may well serve as a guide to our final destination.

I often think about near-death survivors recounting their experiences. They speak of traveling through a tunnel toward a bright white light... similar to the experience of a baby traveling through the birth canal to the light. Does one transition have to do with the other … birth and rebirth?

When I was with Nana during her final hours, she began regressing to a time 70 years prior when she was walking down a street lined with beautiful Cherry trees in full blossom. Even though it was winter, I did not question it. I supported her as I envisioned everything she was experiencing. Don't correct someone who is taking their last stroll down memory lane; just support them and embrace the wonderful opportunity to step out of the world of reality.

There are two things people are anxious about when they die; being in pain and being alone. Thankfully there are many medications available for pain. For those in absence of family or friends, there is a movement spreading to American hospitals to make certain no one is alone at the time of their passing. The attendee is a caring person trained to know what is happening and how to anticipate one's needs.

There are also hospice programs to assist care receivers and their families; as well as to be with the terminally ill who are alone.

We must remember that although medical institutions are capable of providing necessary medical care to the dying, during the final days and hours of life they cannot always provide human presence.

We also need to keep in mind that some people prefer to have their final moment without the presence of those closest to their hearts.

We have all heard about the family members that sat vigil for days, went for coffee, and returned to find their loved one passed during those few moments of absence.

Sometimes the patient will give you a sign that this will be the last goodbye. While preparing to leave from a visit with my aunt during her last days, she asked me to take home a special stuffed animal I had given to her months prior which had a significant meaning to us. I knew something was happening, but I couldn't put my finger on it at that moment. After our kisses and goodbyes, I looked back into her room at the nursing home. In her frailty, with all her might she mustered up a big, courageous full arm wave like a queen ... along with a valiant smile. I gave a gallant wave back saying "I love you", realizing I would never see her again. I lovingly accepted that my aunt wanted to do it her way. Hours later she passed in the company of her favorite aide.

We need to allow the patient the choice of their closure without question.

We need to allow the patient the choice of their closure without question. It is each dying person's unique and individual experience. We are observers. We need to be very cognizant as to their subtle hints and gestures without question or challenge.

No matter who, no matter how, no matter what ...

No one should have to die alone.

In Conclusion

Life is too short. As we look back, it passes swiftly before our eyes.

Why is it that it takes a milestone birthday, the loss of a loved one or the unexpected terminal illness to open our eyes and re-evaluate the choices we've made and how we have conducted our lives?

Now is the time to make the changes; not when, but now. Not if, but how. How can we change today, the now, the present, to make our life what we want it to be?

We are all entitled to enjoy peaceful, loving lives and experience the freedom to make wise choices; to love ourselves free of worry and fear of what others will think.

This is *our* journey, *our* life and *our* death. For if we can be happy, feel settled and be at peace within ourselves, we will have a much better chance of Dying without Crying.

Do Not Stand By My Grave And Weep

Do not stand at my grave and weep,

I am not there, I do not sleep.

I am a thousand winds that blow.

I am the diamond glint on snow.

I am the sunlight on ripened grain.

I am the gentle autumn rain.

When you wake in the morning hush,

I am the swift, uplifting rush

Of quiet birds in circling flight.

I am the soft starlight at night.

Do not stand at my grave and weep.

I am not there, I do not sleep.

Do not stand at my grave and cry.

I am not there, I did not die.

~ Mary Frye